Overcome Fibromyalgia For Life

How To Live Your Life Pain Free And Break Thru The Fog Of Fibromyalgia

By Dr Brad Turner

Disclaimer

This book is intended to be a general guide, to raise awareness, and to help people make informed decisions in the context of their own personal circumstance. As everybody's circumstances are different, so are the remedies you should seek. While many of the recommendations in this book can be applied by almost anybody regardless of their conditions they are not intended to and should not be relied upon to replace personal medical advice.

The author accepts no responsibility for any loss or injury, be it personal or financial, as a result for the use or misuse of the information in this book. If you have any doubts or concerns after reading this book, please speak to a doctor or other qualified person before taking any actions.

From The Author

Thank you for taking the time to read this book. As an author, I understand the importance of creating books which my readers will find both enjoyable and informative. If you have the time and feel generous, please don't hesitate to leave an honest review of this book.........Dr Brad Turner.

Contents

Introduction

Fibromyalgia is a debilitating condition. Once your doctor diagnosed you with this disease, it can come with years of suffering if failure to treat adequately. In some instances, while the doctors try to identify your illness you may continue to experience the pain just like so many others, well this book is for you. It describes every part of the ins and outs of this disease in a way that you can easily relate to and understand. It also shows you ways to counter the problems associated with your illness and how to fight back.

Often Fibromyalgia shows many different symptoms, but with the use of this book, you will manage a way to move forward to overcome your problems. Sometimes, all you need is a little knowledge and with that purpose in mind, I have devoted the book to readers like you, who are suffering unnecessarily. By reading my book, you can find solutions, without too much reliance upon medication or always searching for the right medicine.

At times, doctors maybe baffled by the array of symptoms that come together to make up fibromyalgia so this book gives you alternatives which you can use in conjunction with your doctor's advice, to help rid yourself of the suffering you have endured for a long time.

Although people see fibromyalgia as an offshoot of arthritis or as being associated with other inflammatory diseases, with a little alternative treatment – as outlined in this book –

you can put this all behind you. As you learn more about your illness in this book, you can move on to a triumphal lifestyle that doesn't let the label of "fibromyalgia" get in the way of your happiness and peace of mind. What you are buying when you purchase this book is a solution that works for everyone. That's a valuable asset to have in your fight against this disease.

Fibromyalgia means a variety of different symptoms, some classic, some very misunderstood. The book author realizes that every case is different but that the seriousness of the illness is not diminished just by having manifested itself in different ways. For some, pain thresholds are also very different, and each reader will find and answer which applies to their personal experience of fibromyalgia. What you take away at the end of this book is the ability to cope with any manifestation the illness presents.

The use of self-help solutions, in conjunction with traditional methods, puts you very much in control of your disease and once you get the upper hand over this condition, the pain will naturally diminish. While trying to understand all the causes of this, the traditional approach and the self-help alternative choices, your knowledge and practice will enable you to enjoy in a much more active way.

Within the chapters that follow lie all the secrets experienced and understood by the writer and the medical field on fibromyalgia. Putting the pieces together will free you from the misery and allow you to begin to enjoy life and all it offers. Saying goodbye to the pain of fibromyalgia is likened to saying hello to a new you and that's the first step in the right direction!

Chapter 1
What is Fibromyalgia?

Fibromyalgia Syndrome – commonly known as Fibromyalgia – is a chronic illness typified by pervasive pain, widespread tenderness, fatigue, sleep disturbance and psychological distress. Unlike other disorders, its etiology remains unknown.

The name of a disease was derived from the Latin terms fibro (meaning fibrous tissue), myo (meaning muscle) and algia (meaning pain.)

Many consider Fibromyalgia as a condition similar to arthritis; however, it is not really a type of arthritis. It is comparable though, because it is classified as a rheumatic condition. This means it causes pain and affects the joints and soft tissues. At the same time, it causes pain and fatigue, apart from interfering with the person's daily activities.

Despite its similarity with arthritis, Fibromyalgia is different because it does not damage or cause swelling to the muscles, joints and nearby tissues. However, it often co-occurs with rheumatic conditions such as Rheumatoid Arthritis, Ankylosing Spondylitis and Systemic Lupus Erythematosus.

Chapter 2
Fibromyalgia: Facts and Figures

According to the National Fibromyalgia Association, the prevalence of the condition is pegged at 3-6%. As of latest data, an estimated 200 to 400 million individuals are afflicted with this common disorder – with 10 million living in the United States.

Fibromyalgia is commonly diagnosed in ages 20 to 50, with the incidence increasing in age. In fact, 8% of people aged 80 years and above possess the symptoms of Fibromyalgia, as stipulated by American College of Rheumatology.

When it comes to gender, Fibromyalgia is more common in women. The ratio of female to male sufferers is 7:1, with 75-90% of the entire population being comprised of female patients. Although this is the case, men and children, regardless of ethnicity, can be afflicted with Fibromyalgia as well.

Fibromyalgia is a hereditary condition, meaning it runs in families. If your grandparents, parents, aunts or uncles are diagnosed with this illness, there is a chance that you might develop it too.

Fibromyalgia patients get confined at least once in three years. It results to 5.5 million ambulatory care visits annually. The average yearly cost of the disease ranges from $3400 to $3600, with costs shooting up to as much as $6000.

Because of the symptoms associated with Fibromyalgia, patients miss an average of 17 days of work, compared to other individuals who only use an average of 6 leaves. Because of this, Fibromyalgia-afflicted individuals suffer from a lower quality of life (4.8 out of 10) and loss of work output.

Consequently, its bothersome symptoms make the patients likelier to develop depression (3.4 times more than 'healthy' individuals.) As such, out of the annual Fibromyalgia-caused deaths of about 23 per year, some are caused by suicide. This adds a straining number to Fibromyalgia mortality, with the bulk usually caused by related injuries.

Chapter 3
What Causes Fibromyalgia?

Even in this modern day and age, the cause of Fibromyalgia remains unknown. However, there are some bodily changes and environmental triggers that seem to cause this debilitating disease.

- **Anomalous Pain Perception**

  One of the most prevalent theories regarding Fibromyalgia is abnormal pain messaging. It is said that individuals who develop this condition have a 'different' way in perceiving pain signals around the body. These are believed to arise following the chemical changes in the Central Nervous System (CNS.)

  After all, the CNS, which is comprised of the brain, nerves and the spinal cord, delivers impulses around the body through specialized cells. When the mechanisms of this system are changed, it can lead to the constant pain associated with Fibromyalgia.

- **Neurotransmitter Imbalances**

  Chemical imbalance is another culprit behind Fibromyalgia. Extensive studies show that those afflicted with the disease demonstrate low levels of serotonin, dopamine, cortisol and noradrenaline in the brain. Low levels of these hormones can precipitate Fibromyalgia, since they play a role in the interpretation of pain stimuli.

Apart from that, these transmitters help regulate bodily processes such as behavior, mood, appetite, stress response and sleep. An upset in these routine activities (such as sleep disturbances and traumatic events) is said to cause Fibromyalgia as well.

- **Stress**

More often than not, Fibromyalgia occurs after stress – whether physical or emotional. In most cases, the individual experiences severe pain after the following events:

  o Surgery

  o Childbirth

  o Injury

  o Infection

  o Problematic/ abusive relationship

  o Death of a loved one

- **Sleep Disturbances**

  As it has been mentioned, sleep disturbances can cause Fibromyalgia.

  Before, sleep problems have been treated as a symptom of the disease, since the pain associated with Fibromyalgia can be severe enough to disrupt sleep.

  But now, studies show that people with disrupted sleep experience worse pain, compared to those who sleep well. In effect, it is believed that sleep problems can lead to the onset of Fibromyalgia.

- **Genetics**

  Like other illnesses, genetics plays a role in the development of Fibromyalgia. With this tendency, certain people can manifest Fibromyalgia after an encounter with certain triggers. With that being said, if you have a relative with this disorder, there is a chance that you might suffer from it too.

- **Related Conditions**

  Your risk of developing Fibromyalgia can increase if you suffer from Rheumatic Conditions, disorders which affect the bones, muscles and joints. Examples of these include Rheumatoid Arthritis, Osteoarthritis, Lupus and Ankylosing Spondylitis.

- **Obesity**

  Obesity is considered the new bane of society. Apart from increasing one's risk of developing cancer, stroke, heart disease, arthritis and diabetes, obesity has been linked with Fibromyalgia as well.

  In a study conducted by Paul Mork, et al, it was noted that women with body mass indices of 25 or more (overweight to obese) have a greater tendency of developing Fibromyalgia. Their risk is at 60% to 70% more, compared to females with normal weight. The risk is further heightened in women who do not exercise, or have a weekly exercise time of just one hour.

Chapter 4
Prognosis of Fibromyalgia

Although Fibromyalgia is a chronic pain condition, its prognosis is generally positive, given the breakthrough strides in diagnosis and treatment. Recent studies show that symptoms remain unchanging for a long period of time. With the help of new approved medications – and exercise – about 25% to 35% report diminished pain and discomfort.

Even with a lot people demonstrating better prognosis, the best outcomes are seen in individuals undertaking a multidisciplinary team approach. Those treated by a physician, mental health and alternative therapy experts – all of whom work towards a comprehensive Fibromyalgia treatment - seem to manage its debilitating symptoms the best.

Good prognosis is also seen in children with Fibromyalgia – even greater than that of adults. According to research, juvenile Fibromyalgia symptoms usually wane in 2-3 years.

Although Fibromyalgia prognosis is generally optimistic, poor diagnosis is seen in individuals with disabilities or life crises. Factors such as depression, pain sensation, sleep disturbances and the inability to work usually lead to poorer outcomes. Additionally, the symptoms of Fibromyalgia might lead to negative behaviors, such as the abuse of sleeping pills, alcohol, caffeine and illegal drugs.

Chapter 5
Symptoms of Fibromyalgia

Fibromyalgia brings numerous symptoms, and they might vary from one person to another. Here are some of the common signs reported by patients:

> ➢ Widespread Pain

The common complaint amongst these individuals is the onset of widespread pain. This discomfort can be felt in numerous parts of the body, although it commonly affects the back or the neck.

Fibromyalgia pain is often unceasing – sometimes the discomfort is lessened, sometimes it feels worse. The characteristic of pain varies. The patient might feel any of the following:

- Mild ache

- Burning sensation

- Stabbing, sharp pain

> ➢ **Extreme Sensitivity**

Another symptom experienced by Fibromyalgia sufferers is extreme sensitivity. These individuals are hypersensitive, that even the slightest touch can lead to pain. This manifestation is called hyperalgesia.

A simple accident, such as hitting your elbow, can lead to a painful sensation that lasts longer than usual. This characteristic, on the other hand, is called allodynia.

Apart from being sensitive to the slightest touch, individuals diagnosed with Fibromyalgia respond adversely to food, bright lights and smoke as well. These sensitivities – although they do not come in physical contact with the person – can lead to the flaring of several Fibromyalgia symptoms.

➢ Stiffness

Stiffness is another sign experienced by patients with Fibromyalgia. Stiffness can be severe, especially if you have settled on one position for a prolonged period of time (say, if you have been sitting on your office chair for the past 4 hours.)

Stiffness occurs in Fibromyalgia because this condition causes muscle spasms. The tight and painful squeezing of these muscles then results to stiffness in several parts of the body.

➢ Headaches

Patients who experience pain and stiffness along the shoulders and the neck are also prone to suffer from headaches. The severity of such headaches can range from mild to severe (similar to Migraine.) At times, headaches are also accompanied by nausea.

➤ Fatigue

Apart from bodily aches and pains, Fibromyalgia is known to bring about fatigue. The associated lethargy can be mild and easy to recover from, to exhaustion comparable to that of the flu. Because of this symptom, most Fibromyalgia patients find it hard to function throughout the day.

➤ Paresthesia

"Pins and needles" – this is just one of the many things that describe Paresthesia, another symptom of Fibromyalgia. Felt in the hands, arms, feet and legs, it brings about a tingling, burning, pricking or tingling sensation. Although it does not cause any pain, individuals who experience this report an itching sensation as well.

➤ Poor Sleep Quality

Even if they have slept well the night before, Fibromyalgia patients often complain about poor sleep quality (described by many as non-restorative sleep.) That's because the disorder can prevent the individual from enjoying deep sleep. This phase of sleep is important, because it enables the body to repair and restore itself.

➤ **"Fibro-Fog"**

Apart from affecting the person physically, Fibromyalgia can also disturb one's mental health. This symptom, which upsets learning and thinking (among many other processes), is called "Fibro-Fog."

The "Fibro-Fog" seen in patients is usually manifested by the following:

- Difficulty learning new things

- Memory problems

- Concentration and attention problems

- Confused or slowed speech

➤ **Depression**

Because of Fibromyalgia's effects on the body and the mind, some people develop depression, a condition characterized by helplessness, hopelessness, sadness, and a sudden lost in former interests.

This occurs since Fibromyalgia patients have low levels of certain hormones, which can then lead to depression. In some cases, this mental disorder manifests in people who find it hard to deal with the symptoms of Fibromyalgia.

➢ Anxiety

Anxiety is described as a feeling of worry, fear or uneasiness. While anxiety is a normal thing that most people experience, some find it hard to shrug it off. Anxiety is common in several mental conditions, and it is a symptom for some Fibromyalgia patients as well. Like depression, it can occur because of the imbalance of noradrenaline and serotonin.

➢ Dysmenorrhea

Dysmenorrhea or a painful period is common in women. With the majority of Fibromyalgia patients being female, this has been considered a symptom as well.

The pain associated with dysmenorrhea usually affects the lower abdomen, although it can radiate to the back and thighs as well. The characteristics range from spasmodic to dull yet constant. It can last anywhere from 12 hours to a day.

➢ Restless Legs Syndrome

Characterized as an overpowering need to move the legs (and sometimes the arms,) restless legs syndrome is a nervous system disorder. Also known as Willis-Ekbom disease, this is a symptom for some patients with Fibromyalgia.

Apart from an urge to move, restless legs syndrome also comes with involuntary jerking of the limbs – a sign known as periodic limb movements.

> ➤ **Irritable Bowel Syndrome**

While an entire condition by itself, Irritable Bowel Syndrome is also a symptom for some Fibromyalgia patients. In some cases, these individuals experience stomach bloating and pain. As a result, they can become either constipated or diarrheic.

Chapter 6
Diagnosing Fibromyalgia

Fibromyalgia symptoms – such as pain, fatigue, sleep disturbances and mood swings – are common manifestations. They are so customary that they can be the symptoms of a disease other than Fibromyalgia. Worse of all, the symptoms can come and go through time. Because of these factors, the diagnosis of Fibromyalgia is often delayed. Unfortunately, it can lead to heightened discomfort and delayed treatment on the part of the patient.

If you experience the aforementioned symptoms, the first thing your doctor will do is to rule out the presence of other conditions. He might order the following diagnostic tests:

- Complete Blood Count

- Erythrocyte Sedimentation Rate

- Serum Cholesterol

- Serum Calcium

- Vitamin D Levels

- Thyroid Function Tests

- Kidney and Liver Function Tests

Once other possible diagnoses have been ruled out, your doctor will fit your symptoms according to the guidelines set out by the American College of Rheumatology. To diagnose Fibromyalgia, the following manifestations should be present:

- Widespread pain in four quadrants of the body, with a duration of at least three months.

- Associated symptoms such as fatigue, waking up tired, and difficulty thinking.

In the past, the doctors checked the 18 designated points, where pain in 11 of which signifies Fibromyalgia. However, since the pain can be fleeting, the patient might have 11 tender points today – and 8 the following day. Add to that, the doctors were not really sure about the pressure points to check. Since 2010, this diagnostic criteria has been eliminated from the guidelines, although it is used by some practitioners until today.

Because Fibromyalgia co-exists with other diseases, your doctor will check if you have experienced any of the following as well:

- Headaches

- Stress or anxiety

- Jaw aches

- Irritable bowel syndrome

- Difficulty in urinating

The physician will take a comprehensive family history, given that genetics is a factor in the development of Fibromyalgia.

Since diagnosing Fibromyalgia can be difficult for even the most experienced of doctors, scientific innovations have led to what is believed to be an accurate diagnostic exam for Fibromyalgia. Named FM/a, this kit identifies the disease according to immune system markers. At $700 a piece, this exam is not usually covered by medical insurance.

Chapter 7
Fibromyalgia Medications

Pain, fatigue and disturbed sleep are just some of the many symptoms associated with Fibromyalgia. To address these unpleasant signs, patients are usually prescribed with the following medications:

> ➤ **Pain Relievers**

Since widespread pain is the hallmark symptom of Fibromyalgia, most treatments are geared toward pain management. Over-the-counter pain killers, such as Paracetamol, can be enough to relieve mild pain.

However, there are some people who can be resilient to the effects of Paracetamol. For these cases, the doctor might prescribe stronger medications, such as Codeine. Often packaged with Paracetamol, Codeine works by blocking the nerves that send pain impulses to the brain.

Do note that Codeine should only be taken for a maximum of three days. If you still feel pain after three days, make sure to check with your physician.

Another stronger painkiller that is prescribed for Fibromyalgia patients is Tramadol Hydrochloride. It works by altering the chemicals that lead to pain sensation. Available in 50 milligram capsules, it is recommended for moderate to severe pain.

If you are prescribed with stronger painkillers such as Codeine or Tramadol, make sure to heed these reminders:

- It should be taken in caution; avoid using alcohol or operating heavy machinery while under the influence of this drug.

- Make sure to read the drug label and reminders before taking it.

- Do not take any of these with other medicines, unless approved by the physician.

While these are more effective for pain, these medications can be addictive. Additionally, its effectivity might wane as you use it over an extended period of time, so increased doses might be needed in the long run.

When taking these painkillers, know that you might expect several side effects such as fatigue and diarrhea. Most importantly, remember to seek the assistance of the physician before discontinuing the use of this drug. Doing so abruptly might lead to unpleasant withdrawal symptoms.

> **Antidepressants**

Although depression is a symptom of Fibromyalgia, antidepressants are prescribed to address pain issues. After all, low levels of neurotransmitters can lead to the development of Fibromyalgia. Since antidepressants can boost the levels of certain neurotransmitters, pain can be subsequently relieved with these medications.

Apart from relieving pain, antidepressants are prescribed because of its primary mode of action: to diminish the depressive symptoms. Apart from this, they can lessen the instances of sleep problems and fatigue.

There are different kinds of antidepressants used in treating Fibromyalgia. They include:

- **Serotonin Norepinephrine Reuptake Inhibitors (SNRI)**

   Prescribed for the treatment of depression and anxiety, SNRIs prove to be some of the most effective drugs for Fibromyalgia. Two of three FDA-approved medications belong to this bracket, and they are Duloxetine (Cymbalta) and Milnacipran Hydrochloride (Savella.)

   o **Cymbalta**

   Approved by the FDA in June 2008, Cymbalta works by enhancing the level of norepinephrine and serotonin. These neurotransmitters help control pain, as well as improve mood.

   The recommended dose of this capsule is 60 milligrams per day, although the first week is usually started with just 30 milligrams. In case you miss a dose, you need to take one as soon as you can.

Cymbalta can cause stomach upset, so take this medication with meals. Avoid taking alcohol while on Cymbalta therapy, as it might lead to liver failure. Do not stop this drug abruptly, as it might lead to side effects, such as nausea and headache.

- **Savella**

  Approved in June 2009, Savella is a tablet used in adults with Fibromyalgia. According to several studies, use of Savella markedly decreases pain and fatigue in participants.

  Two divided doses should be taken each day, with the first day starting at 12.5 milligrams only. Throughout the week, the dose will be increased to 100 milligrams (50 milligrams twice a day.) While it is the recommended daily dose, your physician might up your intake to as much as 200 milligrams.

  Side effects of Savella include nausea, dizziness, insomnia and hot flushes.

- **Tricyclic Antidepressants**

  These drugs work by increasing the levels of norepinephrine and serotonin. They are prescribed to patients with Fibromyalgia, since these individuals usually have low levels of the said neurotransmitters.

Apart from boosting brain chemicals, tricyclic antidepressants such as Nortriptyline (Pamelor) and Amitriptyline (Elavil) can enhance the effects of Endorphins – the body's natural painkillers. As a result, they work well in relaxing painful muscles.

While very effective, they come with a handful of side effects, such as dizziness, drowsiness, constipation, dry eyes and dry mouth.

➢ Anti-epileptics

Also known as anti-seizure meds, anti-epileptics are also used in treating Fibromyalgia. In fact, the first drug that was approved by the FDA for Fibromyalgia use belonged to this category.

The first approved medication for Fibromyalgia is Pregabalin or Lyrica, which works by decreasing nerve signals. It helps calm over-sensitive nerve cells, therefore providing pain relief in as short as one week. Available in capsule form, Lyrica is taken in two divided doses per day. The recommended dose ranges from 150 to 450 milligrams, depending on the doctor's assessment.

Like other Fibromyalgia medications, intake of Lyrica should not be stopped abruptly. Doing so can lead to stomach upset, sleep disturbances, headaches and diarrhea.

➢ **Neuroleptics**

Also known as anti-psychotics, these drugs are prescribed for the relief of chronic pain. They work like anti-depressants, easing the symptoms of both depression and anxiety – which are some of the many symptoms of Fibromyalgia. They also promote sleep, which can be disturbed in patients suffering from widespread pain.

Neuroleptics that have been studied in many researches include Quetiapine. In a 2012 study published in the Journal of Clinical Psychopharmacology, results show that a dose of 50 to 300 milligrams per day, taken for a duration of 12 weeks, can improve sleep and mood.

Another anti-psychotic used in Fibromyalgia treatment is Olanzapine. A study published in 2006 shows that it is also effective in decreasing pain in Fibromyalgia patients.

➤ Muscle Relaxants

Muscle stiffness and spasms are often experienced by Fibromyalgia sufferers. To address this symptom, the physician will prescribe a muscle relaxant, such as Cyclobenzaprine. This drug then works by stopping painful muscle contractions.

More than just halting muscular spasms, relaxants are now being prescribed because they have been proven effective in pain, fatigue and sleep management.

Chapter 8
Therapy for Fibromyalgia

According to experts, there is no one cure to treat Fibromyalgia. Although medications are effective in decreasing the severity of symptoms, they cannot cure the disease all alone. For this reason, professionals also recommend mind-body therapies, such as those listed below. After all, research shows that these approaches are effective, especially when they are part of multi-disciplinary treatment.

> ➤ **Cognitive Behavioral Therapy (CBT)**

Although it is commonly prescribed in individuals with mood disorders, CBT has been proven effective in addressing pain issues as well. As such, it is currently being used as adjunct treatment for the disorder.

CBT is a goal-oriented form of psychotherapy. It works on the belief that the way you think affects the way you act. Nonetheless, both play a huge role in the way you feel.

Delivered in a shorter term, it can help change behaviors and thought patterns. Although it is mostly done on a one-on-one basis, this form of talk therapy can be accomplished with a group as well.

In a CBT session, you can expect your therapist to help you gain control over your illness. He can teach you about techniques and coping mechanisms that can help you overcome Fibromyalgia.

What's great about CBT is its immediateness, as it can help patients in a span of 10-20 sessions. As established by numerous studies, it diminishes pain and enhances sleep. At the same time, it can lessen depressive episodes and boost confidence.

While it can help Fibromyalgia patients of all ages, its effects are better received by children. Although it cannot cure the individual by itself, using this therapy alongside other treatment modalities (specifically exercise) can help lessen the severity of symptoms.

➢ **Guided Imagery**

Guided imagery is a form of psychotherapy that can help alleviate the symptoms of Fibromyalgia. According to a 2006 study of Menzies et. al, patients who used audiotaped guided imagery reported lesser levels of pain and anxiety.

In guided imagery, your therapist will ask you sit or lie down. To make you feel more relaxed, he will ask you to think of pleasant scenarios. For example, he might ask you to think of a beautiful day at the beach.

Although guided imagery is often led by a therapist, you can do it by yourself with the help of audiotapes.

The efficacy of guided imagery is said to stem from distraction. Instead of thinking about the disorder, guided imagery helps the individual relax. And when he is more relaxed, his pain sensation will be markedly reduced.

➤ Physical Therapy

Physical therapy is a modality that helps heal, prevent and treat diseases and injuries. Although it cannot fully treat Fibromyalgia, it can help relieve pain. By this virtue, experts agree that this type of therapy can help Fibromyalgia patients with their daily struggles.

Physical therapists can teach the afflicted person with the following techniques:

- Proper posture, which can make muscle function more efficient.

- Self-management skills that can address the symptoms of Fibromyalgia.

- Activities that can relieve pain and stiffness.

- Relaxation exercises that can reduce muscle tension.

- Stretching exercises that can enhance muscle flexibility.

- Other exercises that can build strength and improve range of motion.

There are different physical therapy techniques that can help ease Fibromyalgia. The most famous is hydrotherapy, which involves the use of cold packs or moist heat.

Cold packs constrict the blood vessels, thereby lessening inflammation. Moist heat, on the other hand, dilates blood vessels, thereby improving blood flow. With increased blood flow, more oxygen and nutrients are delivered to the compromised parts of the body.

Hydrotherapy also helps eliminate the harmful toxins. As a result, it speeds up the healing process.

Apart from hydrotherapy, other techniques that can alleviate Fibromyalgia symptoms include:

- Deep-tissue massage

- Transcutaneous electrical nerve stimulation

- Stretching exercises

- Muscle strengthening exercises

- Pain relief exercises

Chapter 9
Alternative Medicine Options for Fibromyalgia

According to Fibromyalgia expert Dr. Mark Pellegrino, the key to Fibromyalgia is a balanced treatment approach. That is why apart from medications and lifestyle changes, doctors recommend the following alternative medicine options:

➤ **Yoga**

Yoga is an ancient Indian practice that deals with the mind and body. This form of complementary medicine involves meditation, physical postures, relaxation and breathing techniques. It is an effective health accompaniment, as it is known to reduce pain, depression and anxiety.

With these three being the symptoms of Fibromyalgia, experts decided to study Yoga – and the possible effects it can have for patients. In a study conducted in 2010, Dr. James Carson and his associates proved that yoga can diminish the said symptoms, apart from improving personal function.

The study featured 53 women, where 25 participated in a "Yoga awareness program." A routine session involved 40 minutes of gentle stretching, 25 minutes of meditation, 25 minutes of group discussion, 20 minutes of yoga teaching presentations and 10 minutes of breathing techniques.

After eight weeks of Yoga, the participants showed marked improvements. These women reported less pain and fatigue and better mood, among many other Fibromyalgia symptoms.

➢ **Acupuncture**

Acupuncture is an ancient form of Chinese traditional medicine. It involves the insertion of needles, which target certain points. Used in both the western and eastern medicine, it has been effective in treating nausea and vomiting, among other illnesses.

As of latest research, studies show that Acupuncture is also effective in alleviating Fibromyalgia symptoms. In a 2006 study conducted by Dr. David Martin and associates, results show that those who underwent acupuncture reported lesser fatigue and anxiety - even up to seven months after treatment.

Acupuncture is known to relieve widespread pain as well. After all, the manipulation of inserted needles can lead to the release of endorphins – the body's natural painkillers.

Acupuncture has been known to affect brain chemistry too. It helps alter the release of neurotransmitters, stopping the chemicals that convey pain signals. With this therapy, pain tolerance is improved. In most cases, chronic pain is assuaged for several weeks.

➤ Massage

Massage is a form of alternative medicine that has been proven effective in reducing pain, muscle tension and stress. It involves the physical maneuvering of muscles and tissues. When done correctly, it can increase blood circulation and enhance oxygenation.

With massage, pain and stiffness and diminished, and flexibility is further enhanced. Because of the numerous benefits of massage, it has been widely studied for Fibromyalgia. In 2009, a study established that massage is effective in reducing pain and increasing pain threshold. Additionally, it can help improve quality of life.

Here are some massage techniques that has been known to benefit Fibromyalgia patients:

- Circulatory Massage – Makes use of deep pressure in order to eradicate muscle tension and alleviate muscle pain.

- Shiatsu – Deals with the manipulation of pressure points in the fingers, knuckles and hands. It is effective in relieving pain and relaxing the body.

- Reflexology – A technique that involves the manipulation of hands and feet. It has been known to alleviate pain, enhance sleep, reduce fatigue and improve mental health.

> **Tai-chi**

Tai-chi is an ancient Chinese practice that involves breath control, meditation and strong and gentle motions. It is based on the philosophy that a healthy body needs a strong mind. Throughout centuries, it has been utilized to improve balance, flexibility and muscle strength, among many others.

Today, it is considered as one of the best alternative treatments for Fibromyalgia. After all, it has been proven effective in alleviating Fibromyalgia symptoms – apart from improving quality of life.

Backing this claim is a 2010 study conducted by experts from Tufts University School of Medicine. Throughout the 12 weeks of therapy, the participants practiced the 10 classical forms of Yang style Tai-chi. At the end of the study, the majority of the participants reported lesser pain, better sleep, more energy and finer physical and mental health.

➤ Chiropractic Care

Chiropractic care is a treatment modality that relies on the principle "the body is a self-healing organism." In this discipline, the chiropractor adjusts the spine to treat widespread pain resulting from Fibromyalgia and other conditions.

To date, it is one of the most famous complementary therapies for Fibromyalgia. Apart from relieving pain, chiropractic care has been proven effective in improving ranges of motion, especially along the lumbar and cervical spine.

To maximize the body's curative properties, the chiropractor will apply gentle movement or pressure. In some cases, he will perform high-velocity stretches. Through these movements, he can improve spinal mobility, which might have been compromised or restricted because of Fibromyalgia.

Chapter 10
Lifestyle Changes for Fibromyalgia Management

As it has been said, there is no one cure for Fibromyalgia. Apart from medication compliance, lifestyle changes can help manage the symptoms once and for all. Here are some simple yet life-changing alterations that can reduce (if not eliminate) Fibromyalgia symptoms:

> ➢ **Consume Healthy Food**

A poor diet can worsen Fibromyalgia symptoms. As such, the only way you can be healthy is if you eat a better diet.

To do so, you first need to improve your food choices. Here are some guidelines to remember:

- Eat foods that are high in fiber and low in fat.

- Make sure to eat a lot of fruits, vegetables and grains. After all, they are high in antioxidants that can eradicate cell-destroying free radicals. These elements are particularly important, as researchers believe that oxidative stress can lead to the unpleasant symptoms of Fibromyalgia.

- Make it a point to consume fatty fishes, as they are rich in Omega-3 fatty acids. Not only are they beneficial for the heart, they can reduce swelling as well. Studies also show that these fatty acids can help reduce pain and stiffness.

- Supplementation with Vitamin D can alleviate pain too, as a deficiency in this vitamin can lead to pain. In fact, those who have low levels of the sunshine vitamin have the tendency to increase the dose of needed painkillers. In order to enjoy pain relief, eat Vitamin D-rich foods such as fatty fish, beef liver, egg yolk and cheese.

While there are foods you need to eat, there are some you need to avoid – and they are preservative-laden edibles. Additives such as Monosodium Glutamate (MSG), which are found in Chinese food and sodas, can activate neurons that heighten pain sensitivity. In fact, a study shows that cutting on MSG can reduce Fibromyalgia-associated pain.

> **Exercise Regularly**

According to experts, exercise is a vital component in the treatment of Fibromyalgia. After all, regular physical activity can prevent muscle wasting and reduce pain and fatigue. It has also been known to improve physical and emotional well-being.

With the many benefits of exercise, physicians recommend patients to take part in long-term exercise programs. A good exercise regimen should include aerobics, flexibility programs and strength-training movements.

In Fibromyalgia, the basic program recommended is Graded Exercise. For this regimen, physical activity is gradually increased over time. The program is started with stretching exercises, in order to relax muscles and avoid soreness in the long run.

After this, mild exercise is commenced. Examples of such work-outs include swimming and walking. Use of equipment such as stationary bikes and treadmills are recommended as well. Once you get the hang of the regimen, the intensity of the exercises will be augmented.

➢ **Get Adequate Sleep**

Sleep disturbance is a symptom of Fibromyalgia, largely because pain can disrupt the patient's slumber. In the long run, sleep difficulties can worsen symptoms. In fact, those who fail to get restorative sleep exhibit worse signs.

In order to combat sleep problems that might worsen Fibromyalgia, physicians suggest the establishment of regular sleep routines. To do so, make sure to follow these recommendations:

- Do not drink a lot of fluids before bedtime, so as to eliminate urinating tendencies in the wee hours of the morning.

- Do not eat large meals before sleeping. A light snack, however, can help foster sleep.

- Do not take caffeinated beverages or alcohol 4 to 6 hours before sleep time.

- Do not exercise 6 hours before bedtime, as the adrenaline might keep you up at night.

- Do not take naps in the afternoon or evening, as this might disrupt your normal sleep cycle.

> **Reduce your Stress Levels**

Studies show that individuals with Fibromyalgia respond worse to stressful situations and encounters. Unfortunately, this stress response can worsen the widespread pain you are experiencing because of Fibromyalgia. As such, stress reduction is a good way to alleviate pain and other associated symptoms.

There are many techniques that can help reduce your stress. Good examples include:

- Biofeedback

  Biofeedback is a regimen that helps control involuntary functions such as cardiac rate, blood pressure and skin temperature. The philosophy behind this practice is that by channeling the power of your mind, you can be more aware of your body. As you become more mindful of your body, you get to control your own health. As with other relaxation techniques, this regimen has been proven effective in decreasing pain levels.

Biofeedback makes use of electrical monitoring equipment. The therapist will monitor your heart rate and muscle tension through devices that beep and flash lights.

Once you are hooked to the equipment, all you need to do is perform deep breathing and relaxation exercises in order to control your heart rate and relax your muscles. While you do these, the therapist can monitor your body's response.

- **Meditation**

Meditation is a beneficial relaxation technique that has been used throughout millennia. A popular technique used in Fibromyalgia patients is Mindfulness Meditation. In this practice, a person is aware and unprejudiced of the thoughts that come into his head.

With meditation, a Fibromyalgia patient can enjoy the following benefits:

o Decreased pain. Meditation can lower the levels of the stress-causing hormone Cortisol.

o Better sleep. Research shows that those who meditate enjoy higher levels of Melatonin, a chemical that boosts sleep.

o Enhanced well-being.

➢ Pace Yourself

Pacing oneself is important for people with Fibromyalgia. This means not pushing yourself to the limit. It also means balancing activity with rest.

If you do not pace yourself, your symptoms can worsen. After all, symptoms vary from day to day. For now you might feel good, but tomorrow you might not. Because of this, you need to maintain a good level of activity.

Remember, avoid activities that can push you to the breaking point. Although exercise can relieve symptoms, doing too much can worsen them. If you want to improve, you have to do the right activities at the right level and intensity. In due time, you can gradually increase the force of your activities.

Chapter 11
Support For Fibromyalgia Patients

Do you feel like you are all alone, and that nobody understands you or your condition? You do not have to worry, as there are groups that offer support to Fibromyalgia patients and their families. If you find yourself looking for someone to rely one, these associations can help you out:

> ➤ National Fibromyalgia Association (NFA) - http://www.fmaware.org/
>
> Founded in 1997, the NFA is a non-profit collective geared towards supporting individuals with Fibromyalgia. Interested parties can sign up for free membership. As a NFA member, you can receive the latest updates about Fibromyalgia research and treatment.
>
> The NFA also hosts the annual Fibromyalgia Awareness Day, where diagnosed persons – as well as their families – can participate in dinners, picnics, walks and other activities. It also features conferences, where established experts share their insights about Fibromyalgia. Apart from being a day of fun, this event is also educational, so that other people can learn more about this prevalent disorder.

➤ Fibromyalgia Network - http://www.fmnetnews.com/

Offering Treatment and Research News since 1998, the Fibromyalgia Network has been helping patients for more than a decade. Through this website, individuals can gain access to informative Fibromyalgia articles, as well as the latest research.

The website also provides numerous resources for coping with the disease. Here, visitors can read advice given by experts, as well as consumer alerts for Fibromyalgia treatments.

Most importantly, this website offers access to local support groups. Through the Fibromyalgia Network, you can attend empowering meetings, share your personal insights and listen to the people who have the same predicament as yours.

Conclusion

Fibromyalgia is a rheumatic condition characterized by widespread pain. The prevalence of the disease is 3-6%, with about 200-400 million living with this crippling illness. The disease is most common in women, with the risk increasing with age. About 5.5 million ambulatory care visits are because of Fibromyalgia. Annual hospitalization costs can range from $3400 to $3600.

The cause of Fibromyalgia remains unknown, although there are several theories regarding the disease. According to experts, the disorder could stem from anomalous pain perception, neurotransmitter imbalances, stress, sleep disturbances, genetics, obesity and other related conditions.

Prognosis of Fibromyalgia is generally positive, given the right mix of medications, therapies, lifestyle changes and complementary medical practices.

The common symptom of Fibromyalgia is widespread pain, which can be accompanied by extreme sensitivity, stiffness, headache, fatigue, paresthesia, poor sleep quality, "Fibro-fog," depression, anxiety and dysmenorrhea. At times, it is manifested by Restless Legs Syndrome and Irritable Bowel Syndrome.

Fibromyalgia is diagnosed if the individual meets the guidelines set by the American College of Rheumatology. They are widespread pain in the body's four quadrants, and the onset of fatigue, sleep disturbance and other related symptoms.

Several medications are used to treat Fibromyalgia. They are painkillers, anti-depressants, anti-epileptics and neuroleptics.

Therapies are also prescribed for Fibromyalgia management. They are Cognitive Behavioral Therapy, Guided Imagery and Physical Therapy.

Alternative Medicine Therapies are also used in conjunction with the aforementioned Fibromyalgia treatments. Proven-effective options include yoga, acupuncture, massage, tai-chi and chiropractic care.

Since Fibromyalgia can be caused by several factors, lifestyle changes are necessary for the long-term management of the disease. Recommended modifications include a healthy diet, exercise, adequate sleep, stress reduction and proper pacing.

For Fibromyalgia support and latest information, patients and their families can visit the websites of the National Fibromyalgia Association and the Fibromyalgia network.

Other Books By Dr Brad Turner

Natural Remedies For Beginners

Discover the key ingredients necessary to lead you to a healthy life. Inside this easy-to-read guide is a plethora of information at the ready to guide you through the process of healing many of your ailments and troubles. You will find natural remedies for anything from insomnia to a sore throat within this manual and will have the tools necessary to combat many of the illnesses that are the result of an unhealthy lifestyle.

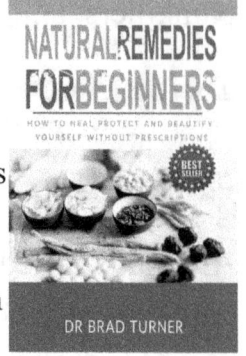

Healing Honey For Beginners

This book is a complete guide for the people about honey and its several uses so that they can make the right decisions depending on their needs and stay thoroughly informed about the various benefits of honey.

Healing Honey For Beginners For Beginners encompasses every aspect of honey starting from the history of honey and humans till the delicious recipes it can be used to make. The book gives a very thorough description of the difference between honey and cane sugar. It has also successfully brought together information on the varieties of honey. For people who are unaware of the true meaning of raw honey, this book can be a great help. Furthermore, the book has complete information on the various forms of honey and which kind of honey can be used for what purpose. It has genuine description of the nutritional facts about honey along with the how to harness honey's health benefits.

Natural Antibiotics And Antivirals For Beginners

Herbs were among the first providers of medicines that had been used by our ancestors thousands of years ago. If anything, they can still be the most convenient sources of medicines.

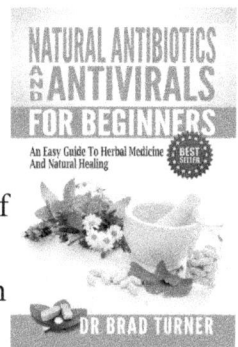

This book is a record of the various medical herbs and their properties. It also entails the preparations of the medicines from these herbs. Herbal medicines have the capacity of curing infections and diseases in the most convenient way. Not only that, but they are also almost completely harmless and have no side-effects whatsoever.

Aromatherapy The Beginner's Guide

Who knew that these are five of the must have essential oils? Dr. Brad Turner does—and we are blessed that he's chosen to share his knowledge and expertise in his latest book, ESSENTIAL OILS. So much has been written about using oils: as cures for everything from toothaches to acne; aromatherapy and even taken internally for whatever reason is popular that day.. To our own peril, we've discovered much of this information is false. Dr. Turner gains our trust immediately with his treatise: never ingest these essential oils. And that's the beginning of an author/reader relationship that will stand the test of time…and information, because Dr. Turner tells the truth. And that's the way we like it!